the

OPTICIAN'S QUICK STUDY

A Simple Skills Guide to Becoming &
Remaining a Great Optician

M. M. CORNELIUS

1

the

OPTICIAN'S QUICK STUDY

This book is not intended to diagnose, prevent or even treat diseases nor does this book guarantee any success you may have using the information and techniques. This book is solely based off of the experience of a certified Optician as she shares her knowledge that she has learned in the field to others in a handy guide. It doesn't replace a full education or apprenticeship in Opticianry.

This is a work of nonfiction. Any procedures and practices in this book should be done with consistency and in compliance with current, professional standards and for individual situations. Although efforts have been made to ensure the accuracy of the contents of this book, the authors, editors and publisher cannot and will not accept responsibility for errors or exclusions for the outcome of presented material. There is no expressed or implied warranty of this book or information imparted by it. Readers should carefully review all materials and literature themselves and be aware of any policy or governmental or changes in law regarding current standards in Opticianry or anything medical or healthcare and optical related while not relying on this book for anything at all. The author, editor, illustrator, publisher or anyone is not liable for anything. Read and study at your own risk.

the OPTICIAN'S QUICK STUDY

*A Simple Skills Guide to Becoming &
Remaining a Great Optician*

Table of Contents

RETAIL SALES & CUSTOMER INTERACTION

Opticians are specialists at eyewear sales, customer service interactions as well as the complete inspection of eyewear prior to the delivery of the eyewear to the patient or patron. In order to become and remain a well rounded and great Optician, one must become a knowledgeable eye care professional by learning the fundamentals of eyewear sales, customer interaction and eyewear inspections. Therefore, the first interaction most Opticians will have is with the patient or patron, and it is during this interaction that the Optician must begin earning patient trust, not losing it.

Earning Patron Trust

Great Opticians are empathetic. They are able to place themselves in the shoes of patrons in order to understand them and their various walks of life and careers. Being empathetic and bringing the knowledge of solving various vision issues with eyewear is at the core of what being an Optician is all about.

Therefore, below are some items that Opticians must provide upon first greeting and maintain throughout their encounters with various patrons in order to begin earning patron trust.

- Smile
- Be Courteous
- Listen
- Clearly Communicate

While providing patrons with the four items listed above, Opticians must also constantly calculate how everything learned from the patron about their way of life will manifest itself in the perfect pairs of eyewear for their daily living. Opticians do this by:

- Asking Proper Questions

- Observing
- Clearly Explaining Benefits of Specific Lenses and Frames
- Persuading with Facts

By providing the patron with the attention required with all of these items, patrons are more apt to engage and trust the lead of the Optician who is interested and cares about their livelihood and long term visual health.

Smile, Be Courteous & Observe

Beginning a conversation with a smile and eye contact is necessary for any Optician because not only does it create a path for easy dialogue, but one can gain much knowledge about current eyewear and eyes by making eye contact. This first contact provides the first details about a patron. An Optician can tell the approximate age, whether the patient has ocular deformities, and if looking close enough, can easily spot if the patient is a contact lens wearer.

Other items that an Optician can learn during conversation are if the patron strains while shopping or reading, how they generally stand, walk and hold their neck and head naturally. These are a few items that will help guide the Optician when fitting the patron with new eyewear.

Listen, Ask & Clearly Communicate

The most important skill an Optician has during communication is listening, and the second most important skill is asking the proper questions. Many times, Opticians will have patrons who don't know where to begin or what to discuss, especially if it is a person who is new to eyewear and vision changes. Therefore, in the event that patrons aren't lifetime eyeglasses wearers with some knowledge base about their preferences, Opticians must prompt with questions, many times explaining clearly why they are asking.

Questions that Opticians should ask will be open ended that navigate the patron to discuss the typical workday, weekend and evening life, from career to extracurricular hobbies and activities, from contact sports to sewing. Knowing the professions and hobbies of patrons assists Opticians in preparing uniquely functioning pairs of eyewear.

Persuading the Patron

The art of persuasion is critical in the sale of eyewear. The Optician is to persuade through a combination of things that include:

- Facts
- Patron's personal style
- Necessity
- Goals

Never persuade with price. Price is never a great tool to use when persuading a patron into the best pair of eyewear for their needs. Although it may seem important, seven times of ten, it isn't as important as one may think. In fact, once most patients understand the reasons behind why they need a specific type of eyewear and how specific lenses and frames can benefit them, they are willing to care for their vision in the best way they can, regardless of the price.

Facts & Necessity

The reason persuasion is necessary in Opticianry is to debunk specific myths and fallacies about selecting and wearing eyewear and lenses. Persuasion has nothing to do with fabricating, or lying, to the patron. Opticians should be armed with the necessary facts, verbally and visually, possibly in pamphlet form as well as through demonstration, in order to erase any apprehension with each patron who has possibly learned alternative, slightly skewed versions of facts about eyewear.

Once an Optician arms the patient with facts through clear communication both visually and verbally, the patient can and will make an informed decision for his or her own being. At this point, the patron isn't being told what to do, but is in control and making the decision all on her own through factual, necessary persuasion.

Style, Goals & Patient History

Other ways Opticians are to persuade patrons are through the patron's personal style and goals. It's vital for patrons to feel excellent while wearing eyewear, and it is the responsibility of the Optician to introduce the most up-to-date eyewear fashions which will complement the patron.

A common way Opticians do this is through the patron's facial shape and structure, balancing it to a particular frame and rim shape as seen below:

<u>Facial Shapes</u>
Round
Square
Oval
Heart
Triangular

With these facial shapes, or structures, the general rule is to go opposite, or move away from frames with rims that match the facial shape. This is the general rule of styling in fashion, and it is to gain and evenness. An oval face probably should not wear an oval frame because the idea is to even the face out, not make it even more oval or elongated.

- Round faces should go with a boxed look - square or rectangle frame.
- Square faces should go circular or oval.
- Oval faces usually look great in a variety, but shouldn't wear oval.
- Triangular faces need a frame to bring balance, or more squared, to the top in a bolder way.

Utilize this knowledge of frame and facial shapes in order to not waste time on the retail floor by having the customer try on styles aimlessly. Instead, have clear targets in mind when you select the frames for your customer to try on based on his facial structure as well as style which you discovered through asking, inspecting the current pair the customer is wearing or introducing a new, trendy style that would look great on the patron's face and be useful in his day to day activities and career, boosting overall confidence.

Finally, the most important items used to satisfy patrons with proper eyewear during the initial engagements are their vision goals and the patron's history. Vision goals must be met as much as possible with each pair of eyewear prepared for the patient. Everything from the doctor's prescription to the style and fit of the frames and lenses are unique to each patient. All of these items are tailored to meet the patient's vision goals.

Some of the questions to ask patrons in order to obtain their unique vision goals have to do with their past and even present such as:

- career/occupation
- hobbies/sports
- previous ocular surgeries
- current visual or ocular issues
- present eyewear

Career, Occupation, Hobbies and Sports

A person's career or occupation reveals where he or she will wear eyewear for at least half of the twenty-four hour day. Therefore, the eyewear must provide optimal vision during the course of the day as well as fit comfortably, without the pain of being too tight across the bridge of the nose, the sides of the nose or behind the ears or on the sides of the face, all of which can become a hassle, creating undo stress related issues for the wearer.

Also, depending on the patron's career or occupation, the eye care professional must fit the patient with the most durable frames and lenses. For instance, if the patron has a history of being rough with frames, frames with flexible temples or more durable frames that can handle a great deal of wear without breaking as easily can be suggested.

Here are just a few familiar frame materials and types in which Opticians need to be familiar:

- Plastic – plastic frames are hypoallergenic, adjustable with light heat using a heat warmer
- Metal – mostly made with nickel and can cause a allergic skin reaction

- Titanium – hypoallergenic, corrosion resistant, very durable and very light weight

Can you see why knowledge of patient history will be valuable when selecting frames? Knowing if a person has metal allergies, an Optician should guide the patron to frames that are hypoallergenic. If a patient has a high minus prescription leading to bulky edges on lenses, the Optician may persuade the patient to hide some of that thickness with a plastic frame.

The same type of knowledge that Opticians need to have for frames goes for lenses as well. One wants to fit a patron with the strongest and lightest lenses, sometimes along with an added antireflective coating or even lenses that transition, depending on the patron's career. One example would be someone who works in construction. It would be a great idea to persuade the patron into polarized, safety standard lenses to protect his eyesight from harmful ultraviolet rays during the day and, at the same time, protect his eyes from impact injuries that may occur from flying debris. This type of safety thickness protection is provided when the lenses are ANSI Z87 standard with verification markings on the lenses upon completion.

Become familiar with all the various types of lenses and their uses, along with the various tints and coatings that can be useful for people working various careers. Next are some examples of various types of lenses, some which are better for specific occupations and hobbies than others.

- Plastic – the basic lens is CR-39 grade plastic and doesn't come with any added benefits. Any extras, such as ultraviolet radiation protection or colors will be added to it through tinting.
- Polycarbonate – the benefits of polycarbonate lenses are that they are light weight and thinner than plastic while also being automatically ultraviolet radiation protected and more shatter resistant than plastic.
- Polarized – These lenses are ultraviolet radiation protected and cut down blinding glare from the sun while also available in a variety of colors. These sunglasses

lenses are great because when indoors, wearers can see just as clearly as if they had on a clear pair of lenses.

- Glass

Of these lens materials, there are specialized lenses, such as Trivex which is a thinner polycarbonate lens. There are also Transition lenses that transition to sunglasses when in the sunlight and transition back to clear when indoors.

Ocular Surgeries & Diagnoses

Opticians may encounter patrons who may have been diagnosed with an ocular disease of some kind, however, aren't fully aware of the way that ocular diagnosis may affect their vision, despite correction with eyewear. This is why it is important for Opticians to be familiar with the general aspects of ocular diseases and even surgeries which may have an impact on how well patrons can see through their eyewear. This comes with the patient or patron history, especially if the

Optician works directly with an Ophthalmologist for prescreening purposes in a medical setting.

The following are some of the common ocular diseases or surgeries that every Optician may want to have a general idea about, especially upon fitting and dispensing eyewear in the event that the patron continues to have issues with vision after attempted correction with eyewear.

- **Age Related Macular Degeneration** – when the macula (at the back of the eye in the retina where the rods and cones are located for vision) breaks down and progressively worsens over time, leading to blindness. There is no cure.
- **Glaucoma** – when there is increased pressure on the optic nerve of the eyeball, leading to vision loss, starting at the periphery and moving toward the center of vision. Common treatment is doctor prescribed eye drops in affected eye(s) in order to halt or slow progression of blindness.

- **Cataracts** – a fogging of the eyeball's lens which prevents clear eyesight due to the lens growing opaque over time. Treatment is in the form of outpatient cataract surgery.
- **Amblyopia** – a particular eye has low vision, leading to the other eye being dominant; sometimes termed lazy eye.
- **Dry Eyes** – eyes lack moisture which can be derived from allergies, eye fatigue, straining, thus causing temporary vision loss. Common treatment is very specific over the counter eye drops only recommended by doctor because all moisture eye drops act differently depending on patient diagnosis.

Those are some of the more common eye problems that Opticians will see day in and day out, and patrons may believe it has something to do with the eyewear and not their ocular diagnosis. Knowledge of ocular diagnoses will assist Opticians in gaining more insight to what may be creating the issue other than the eyewear, and in the end, be able to direct all other questions to the prescribing or diagnosing optometrist or ophthalmologist.

Opticians are not to give medical advice, only eyewear advice. Leave all medical advice to the doctors. Opticians are not to direct patients on how to go about living with their diagnosis. The information about any particular diagnosis or medical history is only to be used for the Optician to better understand what may be the cause of visual issues when wearing eyewear if the eyewear passes inspection. The Optician must always refer the patient back to the doctor for further instruction on diagnosis or so that doctor can review the prescription.

PRESCRIPTIONS, LENSES & HOW TO MANUALLY MEASURE FOR PATIENT

There are a multitude of lens choices for patients depending on their need for visual correction. Once the doctor has written the prescription, many times the eye doctor will request the type of lenses preference to which the Optician will adhere. Other times, the Optician will be the sole guide to which eyewear will best fit the patron based on the prescription and the patron's lifestyle.

Understanding the prescription is vital for the Optician because knowledge of the prescription will provide answers as to how the lenses will appear in a particular frame. For instance, **a high plus (+) prescription for a hyperopic (far-sighted) patient will produce lenses with thin edges and thick middle.** This particular prescription would not do well in a semi-rimless or rimless frame.

Meanwhile, **a high minus (-) prescription for myopic (near-sighted) patients will produce lenses that are very thick on the edges and thinner in the middle**. This particular prescription may appear thinner on the edges with a polycarbonate lenses edge polish while being placed inside a stylish, plastic frame to conceal the thickness of the lenses' edges.

Rx	SPH	CYL	AXIS	PRISM	BASE
O.D.					
O.S.					
ADD:			Additional Orders		
			Doctor's Signature		

Doctor's Office, Address, Phone
Hours of Availability

This type of prescription and lenses knowledge will immediately tell an Optician which frame would work well with the prescription versus another. The Optician can then relay this helpful knowledge to the patient who wants to look great with the final product.

Familiarize yourself with the blank prescription pad above. There are variations of this, and some are even written on blank paper, but they all read the same.

- **O.D.** means right eye. Every number written on the O.D. line is only for the right eye.
- **O.S.** means left eye. Every number written on the O.S. line is only for the left eye.
- **Rx** means prescription. **SPH** means sphere. **CYL** means cylinder.
- **Axis** is the numerical angle that the laboratory uses for the cylinder (CYL) which is marked on the lenses during fabrication for patients with a common diagnosis called **astigmatism**. All prescriptions with a degree of cylinder written inside the prescription field will have a number in the AXIS.

  Astigmatism is a refractive error that happens when the lens and/or cornea of the eye are not shaped like a sphere, but a more elongated shape, causing light to hit on two different spots at the retina. (This is explained later in the book)

- **Prism** is measured in units called diopters and is calculated by using the **Prentice Rule**. The equation is **Prism = Power x Decentration in centimeters**, and this equation is used by Opticians to find the amount of wanted or unwanted prism in a pair of eyewear. Therefore, if the eye doctor prescribes prism on the prescription pad, then it is written under the PRISM column in one or both eyes.

- **Base** is the type of lenses curvature, known as base curve. The doctor can see fit to prescribe base curve for the refractive error. The laboratory will select an appropriate base curve for the lenses as well if the doctor doesn't select.
- **Add** is the bifocal power that will be added to the eyeglasses lenses.
- **P.D.** means pupillary distance which is measured with a pd stick or pupilometer. (On some prescriptions, physicians will input P.D., however, Opticians must measure this themselves as well.)

Rx	SPH	CYL	AXIS	PRISM	BASE
O.D.	-0.75				
O.S.	-1.25	+3.00	45		

ADD: +2.50	Additional Orders
	Doctor's Signature

Doctor's Office, Address, Phone
Hours of Availability

The prescription pad above is now filled in with numeric values. The right eye (O.D.) is a spherical, myopic prescription with no astigmatism, thus no axis. The left eye (O.S.) has an astigmatism, meaning it has a cylinder power and an axis. The Add is the bifocal power needed for near reading distance. Add powers are prescribed for patients with **presbyopia,** or the inability to focus on objects within reading, or near, distance due to an individual getting older. Most presbyopia signs begin between middle to late forties and older. Eye doctors will prescribe presbyopic patients an Add, or bifocal power.

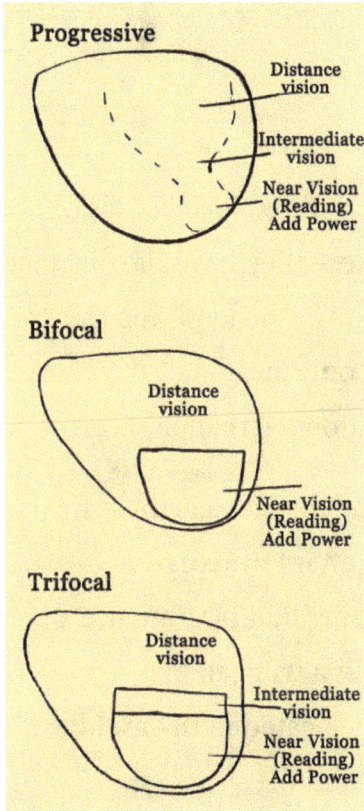

Progressive

Distance vision

Intermediate vision

Near Vision (Reading) Add Power

Bifocal

Distance vision

Near Vision (Reading) Add Power

Trifocal

Distance vision

Intermediate vision

Near Vision (Reading) Add Power

There are various types of lenses that come with an add power. Lenses that don't have an add power are called **single vision**, meaning there is one power throughout the whole lens. Lenses with an add power are called **multifocal lenses**, and these include:

Bifocals (line, round or no-line/blended)
Trifocals
Progressive

Multifocal lenses contain <u>two or three fields of vision</u>. For **bifocals** – bi meaning two – they have the distance vision portion located at the top of the lens, and the near vision which is normally only located at the bottom, minus special occupational circumstances.

   Trifocals – tri meaning three – has three fields of vision – distance, near and an intermediate. Intermediate vision is for reading that is at an arm's length or computer distance. In a trifocal, the intermediate distance vision is located in the middle of the lens between the distance and the near.

   Multifocals are available in line or no-line. Line bifocals/trifocals refer to the line, or segment, that is clearly visible on the front of the lenses whereas no-line bifocals/trifocals don't have a visible segment depicting the reading area.

Progressive lenses are lenses that have three fields of vision that look like they are single vision lenses but are really multifocals. The distance field of vision is located at the top, intermediate the middle and the near at the bottom. Unlike with line bifocals and trifocals, progressive lenses have a narrower vertical field of vision, meaning the periphery of the lenses will become blurry, or less clear.

Though progressive lenses are outstanding when used properly, the Optician must teach the first time progressive lenses wearer how to use them correctly. Line bifocals and trifocals are easier to use because the change in fields of vision is clear to the patient because they can actually see the segmented bifocal in a specific place. However, with progressive, this isn't so. With all multifocal lenses, the patient must drop his eyes and not his head to read. However, with progressive lenses wearers, their eyes must drop <u>in proper alignment with the narrower field of vision</u> than the line bi and trifocal.

For the novice, wearing progressives can take some practice, therefore, Opticians must be thorough in their explanation on how to use along with expectations in the first week to two weeks of wear. Some of the items that could bother the patient are listed below:

- blurry vision when looking to the side with their eyes instead of turning their head
    - Solution: Advise the patient to point their nose at what they are looking at instead of turning their eyes. This is so their eyes remain in the narrower field of vision of the progressive lens

- Blurred vision when looking through the center of the lenses.
    - Possible solution: Adjust the frame on the person's face. When fitting a patient for any multifocal, Opticians must fit the frame to the patients face for comfortable wear. This requires asking the patient how they plan on wearing the frame and what is most comfortable on her face, adjusting the temples, ear pieces and even nose pads, in order that the

measurements for the field of visions in the multifocal sit in the proper area for the unique patient.

- o Possible Solution #2: Double check the prescription, possible unwanted prism, swirls and other defects in lenses.
- o Possible Solution #3: Change the type of lenses for patient because the patient simply can't adjust to the gradual fields of vision after a week or two of wear.

All of these are possible solutions for the progressive lens wearer, however, if the patron cannot adjust, it is more than likely the patient will opt for a blended or line bifocal or trifocal.

What Exactly Is Astigmatism?

Astigmatism happens to be one of those long medical words describing how the light lands at the retina due to either a distorted cornea or a toric cornea. Unless the cornea of a person's eye is spherical, as in a baseball, well, the patient may have an issue of astigmatism because the cornea will have the shape of a football called toric. Torics have two curves and this is what you will see if you inspect a football. Upon a cross section of the football, there is a long curve and short curve. It isn't as a sphere shape where no matter how you cut, inspect, toss, or roll.

This football shaped, or toric cornea, causes incoming light that is needed for eyesight to refract, or bend, onto different areas at the retina, thus, **there isn't one single focus point as there would be in a spherical, smooth cornea, but two** - two curves, thus two focal points at the retina. This will cause any object to be blurry because the light landing in more than one spot at the retina.

Sure, this can be confusing, but just know that unless light is refracted at one spot at the retina, there is astigmatism present, either regular astigmatism or irregular astigmatism. It's all astigmatism! **Irregular astigmatism** is when the cornea has more than two curves, but rather bumpy and totally out of bounds. Light will refract many various ways with irregular astigmatism and it may even require more than glasses or contacts to fix.

Transposing Prescriptions

Eyewear prescriptions are measured in units called diopters. Therefore, the prescriptions written by the doctor are written in diopters, representing the curvature of the lens which gives the optical lens the power that makes the light refract in order to give the patient the best optimal vision possible.

When reading a prescription, an Optician must know how to transpose it as well. Transposing is converting the prescription to another cylinder. When transposing, the numbers may change, but the optical power of the prescription won't change.

Below are the examples and steps in transposing an eyewear prescription. **Remember that the sphere power is always written first, or before, the cylinder power.**

Transposing Prescription with Astigmatism

+3.00 − 4.00 x 90

1. Along the 90 degree axis, the sphere is +3.00.

2. Algebraically add the -4.00 cylinder power to the +3.00 sphere power to get the sum of

-1.00.

3. Add 90 degrees to the 90 degree axis which gives the sum of 180.

4. Change the sign of the cylinder to +

-1.00 +4.00 x 180

Therefore, the refractive error is **mixed astigmatism** because on the 90 degree axis, the sphere is (+) and on the 180 degree axis, the sphere is (-).

Basically, add 90 degrees to the original axis. Then algebraically add the cylinder to the sphere power. Use that sum and make it the sphere power. Then, finally, change the sign on the cylinder.

+3.00 -4.00 x 90 <u>equals</u> -1.00 +4.00 x 180

<u>Transposing a Bifocal to Single Vision Reading Glasses</u>

-0.75 -1.00 x 40   Add: 1.50

1. Algebraically add the bifocal power (Add power) of 1.50 to the sphere power.
2. Don't bother the cylinder or axis.

+0.75 -1.00 x 40

*The axis can never go over 180 degrees. Therefore, if there is an axis of 98, add 90. It equals 188. The axis will be 008.***

Also, Opticians and labs usually work in minus cylinder, while some doctors always work in plus cylinder.

Types of Prescriptions, or Refractive Errors

- A patient who is **Simple Hyperopic** will have a prescription (Rx) that is a (+) sphere. There will be no cylinder, astigmatism and no axis. [+0.25 sph]

- A patient who has a **Simple Hyperopic Astigmatism** will have an Rx that will be plano in sphere and (+) in cylinder with axis.

  [0.00 +0.25 x45]

- A patient who is **Simple Myopic** will have a prescription that is a (-) sphere. There will be no cylinder, astigmatism or axis. [-0.25 sph]

- A patient who has a **Simple Myopic Astigmatism** will have an the Rx will be plano in sphere and (-) in cylinder. [0.00 -0.25 x 45]

- A patient with **Compound Hyperopic Astigmatism** will have plus powers on both the 90 and 180 degree axis, or in other words, the major meridians. Therefore, one must transpose the prescription to this!

  [+0.25 +1.00 x90] and after transposing [+1.25 -1.00 x 180] The spheres are plus.

- A patient with **Compound Myopic Astigmatism** will have minus powers on both the 90 and 180 degree axis. (-) (-)

  [-0.25 -1.00 x90] and after transposing [-1.25 +1.00 x 180] The spheres are minus.

- A patient with **Mixed Astigmatism** will have opposite powers in the major meridians of 90 and 180 degrees. (-)(+) and upon transposing (+)(-).

What Is Base Curve And What Are Laps?

While we are here, remember on the doctor's Rx pad the section for the BASE? Well, the laboratory uses pieces of metal or hard plastic called Laps. These laps all have specific curvatures that suit the eyeglasses prescription. The selection of the wrong lap could mean the lenses don't come out of production as they should. Therefore, the selection of the right base curve lap for the Rx (prescription) is necessary.

Here is a rule of thumb:

The higher the plus prescription, the higher the base curve of the lap.

The higher the minus prescription, the lower the base curve of the lap.

A more average prescription, such as a -1.00 -1.25 x 65, **will take the more neutral base curve of 6** because 6 base curve lap doesn't have a steep curve for a super high plus Rx nor does it have a flat curve for a high minus Rx. It has an average sized curve for an average prescription.

Calculating Prism

What on earth is prism, and how do you calculate it? This isn't a word that most people even say every day, much less calculate. However, as an Optician, prism is something that you must not only know about but know how to calculate. In order to even pass certification or licensing to become an Optician, prism is a topic that won't ever be overlooked as it plays a vital role in how a person sees out of his or her glasses.

What exactly is a prism? Prisms are basically triangular in shape, with an apex (top point or the thin edge on a lens) and a base (flat bottom or the thick edge on a lens). The purpose of the prism is to refract, or in other words bend, where light goes when it enters and passes through it.

As light enters, the light then bends according to the amount of prism ground into the eyeglass lenses. Therefore, the greater strength of the prescription, or stronger the diopters, the shorter the focal length will be.

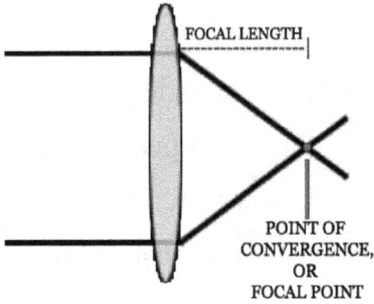

FOCAL LENGTH

POINT OF
CONVERGENCE,
OR
FOCAL POINT

The **focal length** is the distance between the point the light enters the lens to the point where the light converges, or meets, no matter if the lens is plus or minus. The light converges upon entry to a point in the eyeball depending on the strength, or curvature, of the ophthalmic lens.

The strength of the lens is determined by an opthalmologist or optometrist when they use a piece of complex equipment called a phoropter, or refractor. The refractor has lenses of various curvatures that the doctor switches back and forth while the patient reads letters or images from a Snellen Eye Chart during an eye examination. It is from this refraction that the doctor prescribes the patient's prescription in diopters, or in other words, determines the patient's refractive error. Unless an Optician works along side or in a doctor's office, he probably won't see this piece of equipment. Instead, the Optician will receive the prescription the eye doctor wrote to the patient. One can say that Opticians are the "pharmacists" of eyewear.

Back to understanding prism...

Prism in a prescribed lens is used to help the patient gain optimal vision by causing an object that a person is having problems seeing to be brought into focus through the bending of the light. For instance, if a patient is experiencing blurry or unfocused vision, the light isn't centralized in the proper areas on the retina. What using prism will do is help to bend, or refract, the light to a point inside the eyeball which will then optimize that patient's vision. That point is the retina.

With the light being retargeted to the unique focal point for the individual patient, the objects the patient looks at should no longer be unfocused. Prism is generated into the lens in the laboratory based on the prescription.

Now that we know what a prism is and how it operates in lenses to help people see better, how is prism calculated by an Optician?

The Prentice Rule is what Optician's use to calculate prism. The equation was mentioned earlier - **Prism = Power in Dipoters x Decentration in centimeters P=hD**

- P is the <u>prism</u> diopters
- h is distance, or decentration. This decentration is measured in units called centimeters (cm).
- D is dioptric power <u>of the lens</u>

Before moving on, one needs to know and understand the optical center. The **optical center** is the path where the light, no matter its origin at the front of the lens, is supposed to pass without veering another way. If a patient's eyewear contains <u>unwanted</u> prism, the light will pass through on the wrong axis of the lens, not the optical center. This will cause any object that is within the line of vision of the patient to be moved to another position, therefore, causing the patient to not see clearly, or have vision which can result in multiple problems.

Now that we understand optical center, let's say that an Optician needed **to find the prismatic effect of a +6.25 lens at the focal point of 5mm away from the OC, or optical center of the lens.**

The first thing that needs to be done is the conversion of the mm to cm, thus making it .5cm as the equation only calculates in cm. (Optical measurements are always taken in mm so conversion to cm is necessary.) Next would be to plug the numbers into the equation **Prism = Power in Dipoters x Decentration in centimeters [P=hD].**

$$P= +6.25 \text{ x } .5cm$$

P=(+6.25)(.5cm) We are now multiplying D and h.

The prismatic effect [P] = 3.125 D.

Thus P=3.125, and this is how much prism power is in the lens.

Seems pretty simple right? Well, so far, but prism gives some of the most experienced Opticians problems sometimes. This is exactly why there is another way to calculate prism which is through a **manual lensmeter**.

Using this piece of optical equipment allows the Optician or laboratory professional to see just how much wanted or unwanted prism is in the eyewear by counting circles! In order to pass the certification and licensing exams for Opticianry, one would need to know both methods.

With a manual lensmeter, which looks similar to a microscope, Opticians can look inside and see a bullseye with rings called recticles. It is when looking inside the lensmeter that the Optician can locate the optical center easily upon gently placing the eyewear onto the lensmeter. The lensmeter has dials that will be used to match the written prescription.

- The prescription will come in clear as intersecting green lines if the prescription is spherical.
- The lines come in clear separately if the prescription is spherocylindrical, or there is astigmatism.

- If the green lines don't come in clear or at all, the prescription is wrong. The eyewear won't pass inspection.

The optical center will generally be somewhere near the center of the lenses, unless there is some type of strabismus. If the intersecting green lines are too many millimeters off from the OC, the lenses will be considered to have prism. The circular rings away from the center are how many diopters of unwanted prism is in the lens. Therefore, counting them will reveal the prismatic effect and the location of the prism.

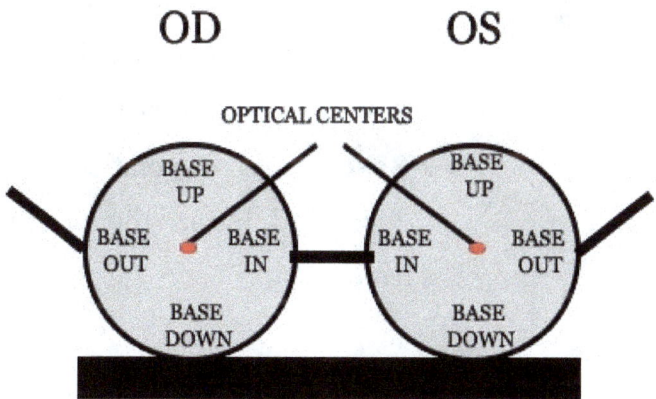

OD   OS

OPTICAL CENTERS

BASE UP

BASE OUT   BASE IN   BASE IN   BASE OUT

BASE DOWN

BASE UP

BASE DOWN

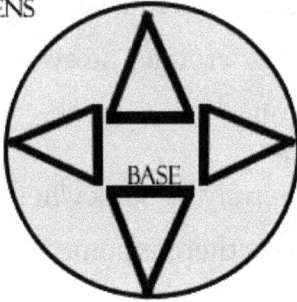

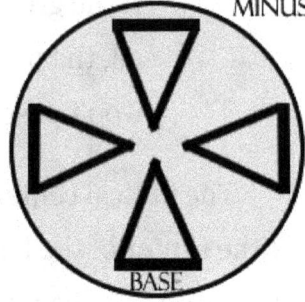

PLUS LENS

BASE

MINUS LENS

BASE

Prism has four different locations. Those locations are based on which lens is being inspected. The four locations are:

- **Base In** – when the prism is going toward the nose
- **Base Out** - when the prism is going toward the ear, or temple.
- **Base Up** – when the prism is upward, toward the upper part of the lens
- **Base Down** – when the prism is downward, toward the lower part of the lens

Lenses are made of prisms. Plus lenses are thicker in the center and Minus lenses are thicker on the edges.

- In plus lenses, the bases of the prisms are toward the center of the lens while the apexes of the prisms are toward the edges. This means that with a plus lens, the edge is thinner, and the center of the lens is thicker.
- In minus lenses, the bases of the prisms, or triangles, are at the edges and the apexes, or points of the prisms, are toward the center. This means that with a minus lens, the edge is thicker, and the center of the lens is thinner.

When placing a lens on the lensmeter, the front of the lens is facing the Optician. Therefore, one must be aware of which lens is being inspected and if the lens is a plus or minus lens. Next, one must read the prescription through the recticle. If there is prism, the clear green lines will be seen a distance away from the optical center on the circular rings.

In the plus lens, which is the right eye if sitting on the lensmeter, the prism displacement (green) is in the direction of the frame's bridge, thus BASE IN. In this case, 2 diopters of base in prism because it is two rings from the center.

In the minus lens which is the left eye, the prism displacement (green) is in the direction of the end piece which, thus BASE OUT. In this case, 2 diopters of base

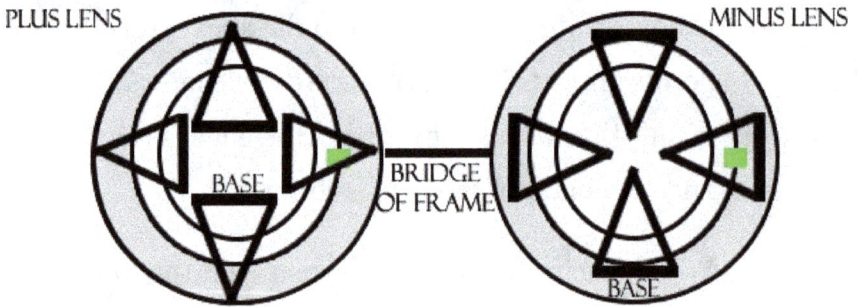

PLUS LENS   BASE   BRIDGE OF FRAME   BASE   MINUS LENS

out prism.

Notice that the green prism displacement is in the same area in the lensmeter, however, two different lenses are being inspected. The plus lens is the OD, or right, and the minus lens is the OS or left. (Remember: When sitting eyewear on the lensmeter, the front of the eyewear faces the Optician.)

Know Your Metrics As An Optician!

Unfortunately, all of the math from middle and high school come into play when an Optician, therefore, one must reach way back and remember simple metric conversions or re-learn all of it. The metric system is the way things are measured in this optical profession across the board. There is absolutely no way possible to obtain success as an Optician without understanding this simple rule of measuring.

The meter is the unit of measure used in any ophthalmic practice. It isn't necessary to learn from millimeter to kilometer, but it is necessary to know how to convert from millimeter to centimeter and back, especially for calculating prism. For now, we will convert from millimeter to meter, just for review purposes. Millimeter is the smallest unit of measure and meter is the standard.

millimeter(mm), centimeter (cm), decimeter(dm), meter(m)

- **Milli – 1000**

- **centi- 100**
- **deci- 10**
- **meter 1**

1.) 2 meters = 2000 millimeters

Solve by multiplying 1000 by 2 or solve by moving the decimal point three places to the right, going from 2.0 to 2000.

2.) 3.2 decimeters = .32 meters

Solve by dividing 3.2 by 10 (because you are moving to a larger unit of measure) or move the decimal point one place to the left, going from 3.2 decimeters to .32 meters.

Remember: When converting from larger unit to smaller unit, move the decimal to the right (or multiply). When converting from smaller unit to larger unit, move the decimal to the right (or divide). Also remember that each unit is separated by 10, so if only moving to the unit next to it, divide or multiply by ten/ move decimal point one spot right or left.

Example of moving the decimal point:
5000 mm = 500.0 cm = 50.00 dm = 5 m

What Are Single Vision Lenses & How To Fit Them On Patient?

Single Vision lenses are exactly what the name states – lenses that have only one field of vision, unlike bifocals, trifocals or progressive lenses which have two or three. Single vision lenses can be used for either distance vision, intermediate vision, or near vision for reading, however, not all at the same time. Measuring a patient for single vision lenses is done as follows:

- Seat the patient directly in front of you.
- Place the adjusted frame onto the patient's face and ask patient to adjust to how they will more than likely wear them.
- Instruct patient to look into the distance, at least twenty feet away.
- You, the Optician, adjust your seat so that you are seated at the same height as the patient.

- Use a permanent marker (Sharpie), place a dot on the lens directly at the patient's pupil. Do this to both eyes.
- Remove the eyewear.
- Measure the height from the bottom of the lens as it sits in the frame to the marked point called the optical center with a PD stick.
- Document this for the laboratory. Don't forget to use the pupilometer to measure the PD (pupillary distance).

How to Fit Patient for Bifocals Manually

All Opticians must know how to measure for bifocals for a patient's eyewear, or eyeglasses, manually and efficiently.

- Seat the patient directly in front of you.
- Place the adjusted frame onto the patient's face and ask patient to adjust to how they will more than likely wear them.
- Instruct patient to look into the distance, at least twenty feet away.
- You, the Optician, adjust your seat so that you are seated at the same height as the patient.
- Use a permanent marker (Sharpie), place <u>a small horizontal line</u> on the lens directly at the lower eyelid of patient or even better from experience, a millimeter below the lower eyelid. Do this to both eyes.
- Remove the eyewear.
- Measure the segment height with a PD stick.

- Document this for the laboratory. Don't forget to use the pupilometer to measure the PD (pupillary distance).

How to Fit Trifocals for Patients Manually

Measuring line, or segmented, tri-focals manually, isn't that much different from the measuring of segmented bifocals. The only difference is where the segment is positioned in the pair of eyewear, or eyeglasses. Opticians must know how to do this manually.

- Seat the patient directly in front of you
- Place the adjusted frame onto the patient's face and ask patient to adjust to how they will more than likely wear them if necessary.
- Instruct patient to look into the distance, at least twenty feet away.
- You, the Optician, adjust your seat so that you are seated at the same height as the patient.

- Use a permanent marker (Sharpie), draw a line on the lens directly beneath (1mm-2mm) the pupil of patient. Do this to both eyes. This is where the laboratory technicians will position the top segment.
- Remove the eyewear.
- Measure the segment height with a PD stick.
- Document this for the laboratory. Don't forget to use the pupilometer to measure the PD (pupillary distance).

In a tri-focal lens, there are three fields of vision – distance, intermediate and near. There will be a two segments, but only the top segment is used for fitting a patient properly for eyeglasses. Therefore, do not take a measurement for two segment heights.

How to Fit Progressive Lenses for Patients Manually

Measuring for progressive lenses segment height is quite different than both the segmented bifocal and trifocal because there isn't a line. The other difference is that the measurement is taken at the pupil. Opticians must know how to do this manually.

- Seat the patient directly in front of you
- Place the adjusted frame onto the patient's face and ask patient to adjust to how they will more than likely wear them if necessary.
- Instruct patient to look into the distance, at least twenty feet away.
- You, the Optician, adjust your seat so that you are seated at the same height as the patient.
- Use a permanent marker (Sharpie), place a dot directly on the lens at the pupil of patient. Do this to both eyes.
- Remove the eyewear.
- Measure the segment height with a PD stick.

- Document this for the laboratory.

Know Frame Measurements & Frame Parts

Opticians are frame experts, and knowing frame measurements are key to dispensing a great pair of eyewear. There are multiple inscribed numbers on a frame. These numbers are the temple measurement, bridge and the eye size, and these measurements are located on the inner portion of the temple and on the inner portion of the bridge.

The eyewire, or the portion of the frame that holds the lenses, must be measured in at least two ways and an optional third. These measurements are the A, B, and ED measurements seen below.

A is the horizontal distance from one side of the eyewire to the other, the longest portion. It is wise to double check this manual measurement with the inscribed A measurement on the frame. This measurement is important to get accurate in order to stray away from unwanted prism as well as the "pulling" sensation caused by unmatched optical centers eyewear to patient.

B is the <u>vertical</u> distance from the top and bottom eyewire, the longest portion. This measurement is important to get accurate in order to prevent unwanted vertical prismatic effects as well as improper bifocal settings.

ED is a measurement that crosses the center of the lens, going from the bottom eyewire to the other side <u>diagonally</u>. Many times, the laboratory doesn't need this measurement, making it optional.

DBL is the bridge width or the distance between the lenses(DBL). This bridge measurement is sometimes inscribed on the inside of the bridge. This measurement is taken at the nasal or at the bridge of the frame between the eyewires. A wrong DBL throws all measurements off in the manufacture of eyewear causing prism and more.

Temple – this measurement is written on the inner temple and it is the largest number. It is the length of the temple that doesn't have to be measured, but read on the frame. Temple length is important for frame fit.

Oh yes, and don't forget the PD or the interpupillary distance measurement. This measurement isn't on the frame however. It is actually on the patient. This measurement can make or break the finished eyewear product as this measures the distance between the patient's pupils with a PD stick or Pupillometer. If this is wrong, well toss the pair of glasses as depending on how off the measurement, any thing from prism to simply can't see is going to be the problem.

One the next page, you will learn the basic frame parts. All Opticians must know the parts of frames as well as how to adjust the frames, depending on their style and material in which they are made. For example, if the frame is plastic, light heat from a **frame warmer** may be necessary to adjust. However, if the plastic frame is very aged and dry, the frame may break upon adjusting because the material has been weakened due to age and wear. An Optician should not attempt to adjust a frame in this condition unless the patron insists and completely understands that the frame may break during adjustment and there is no liability to the retail shop. The better option for the patient would be to purchase another set of eyewear.

As far as metal frame adjustments, a frame that is in good condition should be adjusted, but without a frame warmer. Metal and Titanium frames don't need heat for adjustment. However, all frames, no matter what their make, require specific tools to adjust them for patients and also to display the required **four point touch**.

The four point touch is when a pair of eyewear is on a flat surface and each point on the eyewear touches the flat surface, whether the frame is turned over upside down (the eye wires and the end of the temples are touching the flat surface) or right side up (the temple tips and eye wires touching flat surface).

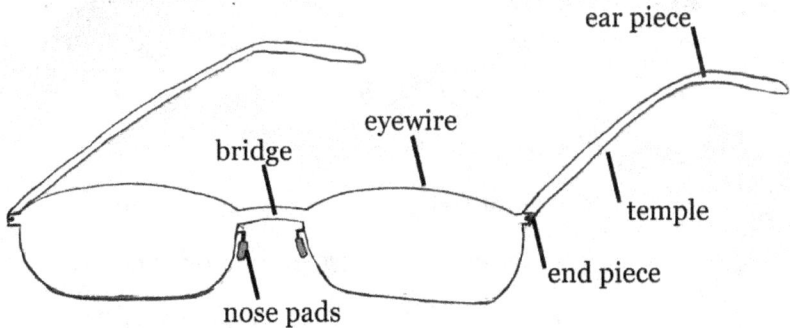

bridge
eyewire
ear piece
temple
end piece
nose pads

Optical Eyewear Adjustment Tools

Confession. Many Opticians use their fingers for simple frame adjustments, however, this shouldn't be the case. There are special tools specific to the parts of frames that need to be adjusted. Some of these tools are listed below:

- Chain Nose Pliers – used to grip and adjust the nose pad arms to make the nose pads fit more snug or loosen them to relieve the pinch from the patient's nose.
- Double Nylon Jaw Pliers – used to grip and adjust without damage major parts of the frame like temples and even the end pieces.
- Screw Driver – used to screw and unscrew screws from the end pieces in order to loosen or tighten the lenses into the frame's eyewire. They are different sizes.

- Nut Drivers – used for tightening and sometimes even loosening nuts and bolts.
- Axis Pliers – used to adjust for lens axis correction where the lens is placed between the rubber portion of the tool and twisted on axis.

What Is a Pupilometer & Why Use One as an Optician?

A pupilometer is a device used in Opticianry that measures the distance between a patient's pupils. It is held by the Optician and placed lightly against the forehead of the patient. Normally, the patient holds the other end for positioning purposes.

Inside is a light to which the patient focuses. The Optician then measures the distance between the patient's pupils with adjustments atop the device. It is with this pupillary distance reading that eyewear can be crafted to fit their individual needs. If the PD measurement is wrong, it will affect how the patient sees through his or her eyewear in a negative way.

Unless the patient has a form of **strabismus**, or eyes that are misaligned, the right and left eyes usually measure the same or within two millimeters when measuring each eye individually.

KNOW THE EYE & LIGHT, LENS MATERIAL

Knowledge of the eye and how it works is crucial as Optician. There are many natural occurrences in the outside world that affect how well eyes operate. One of these natural occurrences is the sun's natural light. It is important to understand what types of light rays affect eyesight and what can be done to minimize harmful effects of light rays on eyesight. Therefore, we will move on to learn about the electromagnetic spectrum.

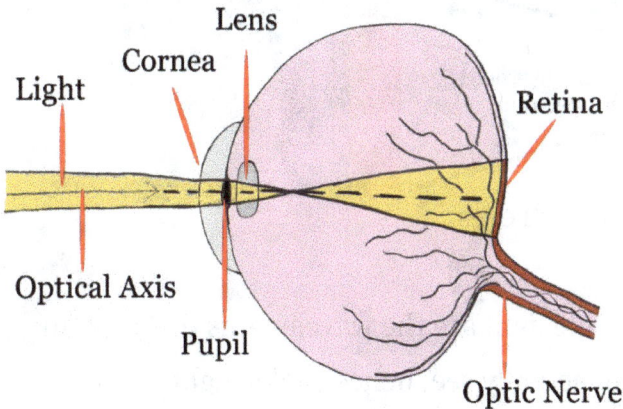

THE ELECTROMAGNETIC SPECTRUM

The electromagnetic spectrum is the full array of radiation, or light, being emitted at all times. There are different types of radiation being emitted, and all of their wavelengths are measured in units called nanometers (nm). Opticianry, as figure 1 below states, focuses mainly on visible light and ultraviolet radiation that enters the eye. What happens to the visible light as it enters the eyes determines visual acuity, or how well

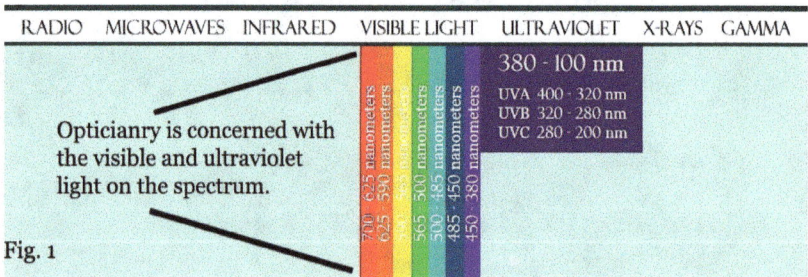

| RADIO | MICROWAVES | INFRARED | VISIBLE LIGHT | ULTRAVIOLET | X-RAYS | GAMMA |

380 - 100 nm

UVA 400 - 320 nm
UVB 320 - 280 nm
UVC 280 - 200 nm

Opticianry is concerned with the visible and ultraviolet light on the spectrum.

700 - 625 nanometers
625 - 590 nanometers
590 - 565 nanometers
565 - 500 nanometers
500 - 485 nanometers
485 - 450 nanometers
450 - 380 nanometers

Fig. 1

vision is in both eyes.

Visible light are the wavelengths that human beings can actually see, hence visible light. This particular section of the electromagnetic spectrum sits between the infrared and the ultraviolet radiation.

Visible light wavelengths range from 380 nm to 700 nm, and they are most important to eyesight.

One of the best ways to think of wavelength is to separate the compound word into two words – wave and length. Now, wave your hand extremely slowly. The length of time it took to get to the other side of the wave was much longer than if you would wave your hand

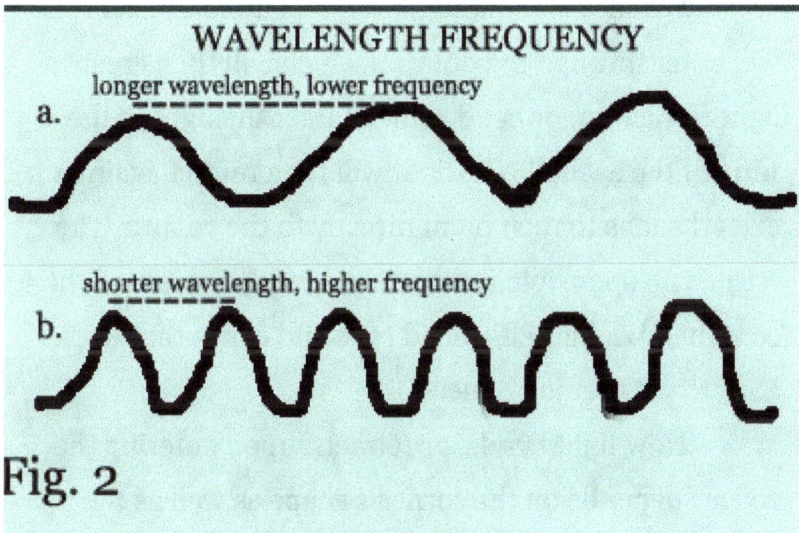

WAVELENGTH FREQUENCY

longer wavelength, lower frequency

a.

shorter wavelength, higher frequency

b.

Fig. 2

faster, or at a faster, higher frequency.

The higher the wavelength frequency, the hotter the radiation and the shorter the wavelength, thus

giving us the change in color that we see if we are examining a flame of fire, for instance, as it goes from orange (hot) to blue (hotter).

Therefore, upon inspection, Figure 2a has a **longer wavelength and lower frequency** than Figure 2b which has **shorter wavelength and higher** (faster) **frequency**. The wavelength is found by measuring the distance between **wavelength crests**, or the top point of one wavelength to the next, as shown by the dotted line.

When this radiation, or light, enters eyeballs, it will enter through the **cornea** which will then create a light refraction, or bend, which target the light to the **lens** of the eyeball. The light will then refract again as it exits the lens to then point directly to the **retina**. The retina is responsible for the colors we see because it has contains specific cells called rods and cones that work hard to get that job done.

How light bends, or refracts, upon entering the cornea depends on the cornea's shape as well as the lens shape and/or abnormalities. Common refractive errors such as astigmatism, presbyopia, hyperopia, and myopia are a direct result of the shapes of the cornea and/or the lens. For instance:

- If the curvature of the lens isn't equal on all sides as a sphere, but more like a football, light will hit different parts of the retina, thus, making way for **astigmatism**, when light hits the <u>front and back</u> of the retina <u>at the same time</u>.

- If the patient has a longer eyeball shape, then **myopia, or nearsightedness**, will occur. This also happens if the cornea has too much curvature. The light entering the eyeball will not focus on the retina, but **in front** of the retina, leading to nearsightedness.

- If the patient has a shorter eyeball, then **hyperopia, or farsightedness**, will occur. This also happens if the cornea does not have enough curvature. The light entering the eyeball will not focus on the retina, but **behind** the retina instead, leading to farsightedness.

It is important for Opticians to understand the reason behind the refractive errors so that they are able to more understand how eyewear has the ability to correct refractive errors. Lenses become the first point of contact for light, thus, the prescription, or curvature, placed into the lens during pre-fabrication and fabrication in the laboratory has the ability to refract the visible light where it should point in the eyeball to hopefully give the patient clear or improve their vision.

Upon assisting a patient, or patron, with eyewear, Opticians must also understand the dangers of ultraviolet rays when those light rays make contact with eyes. There are three types of UV light – UVA, UVB, and UVC. (Refer back to figure 1) Therefore, it is important to know which lenses can protect a patron's eyes against UV damage.

The damage that UV light causes to eyesight are:

- retina damage such as macular degeneration
- lens damage such as with the formation cataracts which creates a translucent lens over time
- photokeratitis, commonly known as sunburn to the eye, where the cornea is inflamed.

Because ultraviolet radiation is ever present, regardless of the season of the year, it is vital that Opticians know which selections of lenses are best for the protection of vision. Opticians should always have the goal of fitting patients with the best protection for their eyes.

SELECTION OF LENSES FOR EYEWEAR

How certain lenses protect eyes from UV light is a necessary characteristic of eyewear that needs to be addressed when persuading a patron in their eyewear needs. The lenses that automatically protect eyesight from UV light are:

- **polycarbonate and Trivex**
- **polarized**
- **Photochromic**, or lenses that darken in the sunlight but become less dark when indoors

UV Treated CR-39 Plastic lenses – these are not automatically UV protected. They MUST be UV treated in order to protect from UV light.

These are lens materials that protect against UV rays completely. Many patients don't realize that a tinted lens doesn't necessarily protect against UV light. It only provides a different color. Therefore, many people are walking round with over the counter sunglasses that have no UV protection. They are only tinted to a darker color. Meanwhile, their eyes are being hammered by ultraviolet radiation during all parts of the day.

The Optician should persuade the consumer through facts that polarized lenses will protect their eyes all year from UV rays, even in the winter, when light reflects from water and snow. An added bonus about polarized lenses is that they can be worn indoors and one can see just fine though the lenses are very dark. Polarized also comes in a multitude of colors from yellow to gray.

Another very important quality of polarized lenses is that they protect against glare from the sun, which can be blinding, especially when driving. A great example of this type of glare is the morning sun or the glare that forces your hand to your eyes at the traffic lights. This affects every driver at one point or another.

Another example of a profession where polarized lenses are a necessity is truck driving. Truck drivers need to protect their eyes from glare and UV rays from all angles because their eyes are constantly in motion, from the center to the periphery. Therefore, a wrap frame with polarized lenses is a must.

For patrons who want complete UV protection coverage, instead of sunglasses frames that sit out from the face, be sure that the sunglasses frames are as close to the face as possible. This is accomplished with a wrap frame. They protect the patron's eyes from the sun well because they fit the face well around the eyes, preventing damaging rays from entering via the top, bottom, and the sides.

An Optician, no matter where he or she works, must know the various types of lenses and frames that best protect the patron's eyes based on that patient's lifestyle. Get to know and learn the various lens options in the laboratory and what specific characteristics each does to **enhance and protect** the patient's eyesight depending on their **lifestyle**. Again, every patron should be persuaded into UV protected eyewear, clear and polarized.

Safety Glasses, Proper Inscription and Thickness

Opticians will encounter various safety glasses needs from patients who work in industries requiring protective eyewear, and some of those patients need prescription safety eyeglasses. Safety glasses must have a safety inscription which verifies to any inspector that the eyewear is of the proper thickness to protect the patient. Safety glasses come with or without side shields, and an Optician must always ask the customer what his work requires.

When the laboratory is preparing lenses for someone who desires safety lenses, the only difference in preparation will be the thickness at the center of the lens which must meet quality ANSI (American National Standards Institute) standards, and the inscription must be visible to the 'naked' eye on the outside of the lenses near the end piece as to not interfere with the patient's vision. The inscription reads Z87. This inscription verifies that is passes inspection for safety eyewear.

Safety glasses can be made as single vision or multifocal. In fact, some patients such as painters, may need a bifocal segment for near vision on top and bottom of the lenses because the painting profession requires near vision below and above. Opticians must not only be able to sell and fit prescription safety eyewear properly, but also obtain information about the patient's occupation that will be best for the job.

Troubleshooting Vision Problems with Prescription Eyeglasses

When a patient or customer returns not satisfied with eyeglasses, complaining of vision problems during wear, the first thing any Optician must do is listen well in order to learn how to troubleshoot the patient's vision problems swiftly and accurately by a list of quality standards checks.

- Review the eyeglasses prescription to be certain the eyeglasses prescription is identical to the prescribing doctor's Rx, taking notice that if the eyeglasses prescription is in the high plus or minus that there can't be too much variation at all in the prescription as this could alter a patient's vision.
- Check the patient's pupillary distance, or PD, with what is marked on the eyewear. If they are at different locations, this could cause a "pulling" or "strain" effect on the person's eyes. The

inset/outset of the lenses in the frame should match with the person's pupil.

- Check pupil height, being certain that it isn't too high or low.
- Check for unwanted prism and waves.
- Check bifocal heights, making certain the bifocal isn't too high or low.
- Check for scratches or swirl marks interfering with vision.
- Check vertex distance and ask the patient at what location is the vision better, closer of further away from the face. Sometimes this can be fixed with a simple adjustment, but other times, the patient needs a change in prescription.
- Check for proper **pantoscopic tilt** which could move the pupil height dramatically.

> Frames don't normally sit straight vertically up and down, but instead have a tilt, the bottom of the frame closer to the face, or cheeks. The top of the frame should be slightly further away from the face. This is called pantascopic tilt. The opposite of this is **retroscopic tilt** when the top of the frame is closer to

the face and the bottom of the frame is further away from the cheek.

- Check with the prescribing physician to find out what the person's best refracted, or corrected, vision is with the prescription. It may not be that the patient is able to see a perfect 20/20, but maybe only a 20/60. Also find out if there are any ocular conditions such as cataracts or recent cataracts removal, macular degeneration or more that could create possible vision difficulties for the patient. If so, simply send the patient back to speak with their Ophthalmologist or Optometrist for further information or a prescription recheck. Do not take on the doctor's assignment and begin to explain a patient's diagnosis. Allow that person to visit their doctor. Use the information obtained about the patient's possible diagnosis for future reference and issues that may arise in the future when fitting them for eyewear.

Manufacturing Errors Commonly Overlooked In Eyeglasses & Lenses

Many Opticians have never worked in a laboratory as a lab technician actually making the eyewear, therefore, some manufacturing errors they can overlook if not paying close attention and will not meet quality standards of inspection prior to dispensing to patients. Below are some commonly missed manufacturing errors made in laboratory to either the frame or lenses prior to inspection that Opticians must check for prior to dispensing for good customer service and customer retention.

LENS MANUFACTURING ERRORS

Scratches

Scratches and more scratches – Okay so there really isn't any need to define what a scratch is because it is pretty much self explanatory. During the manufacturing process or even during dispensing, things happen, and when things happen, scratches on a freshly made pair of eyewear can happen, too.

Whenever inspecting a pair of eyewear, it is crucial to inspect for scratches that are fine or just plain blatant. Reason being is because these scratches have the potential to interfere with vision or in the least worrisome of cases, just make the highly expensive pair of eyewear look tacky. This isn't great customer service. Therefore, search under a lamp for those common irksome scratches.

Prefabrication Swirl Marks

Oh to damnation with swirl marks! It is a wonder how on earth swirl marks even get by undetected before leaving the laboratory. Anyway, lenses must go through a process on the cylinder machine after the lens has the prescription cut or "generated" into it. The reason for this is because the generator, which is the machine used to grind in the prescription, leaves highly defined marks in the lens, so much so that it isn't see through.

Therefore, in order to begin the process of clearing the lens, one must use the cylinder machine.

Swirl marks are fine circles, like circular scribble marks, all over the lenses or in a particular area which will impair the patient's vision. These marks can be overlooked if not paying attention or holding the lenses up to the light for inspection after polishing. Polishing is the final step in clearing the lens.

Pits

Pits may only occur in polycarbonate lenses. Why? Because plastic lenses don't require what is called a coating. Without a coating on polycarbonate lenses, scratches will occur extremely easily, thus the need for coating. However, along with coating application, another issue could result harming the overall readiness of the lens and that is the formation of what is known as a pit.

Pits are small bubbles on the back surface of the lens. Imagine a sink full of water and one very small bubble floating around in it, except for on a lens, it doesn't float but is stagnant and hard. This bubble, or pit, is totally not supposed to be present on finished lenses, and if detected, will cause the entire pair to not meet quality standards.

Chips

Surprisingly enough, chips do get pass inspection to the final pair of eyewear, and many times, it is by pure accident. Chips on lenses can occur upon mounting, or putting the lenses securely inside the frame. The chips occur on the edges of the finished lens, and sometimes, chips can even be hidden with the frame's rim, therefore, it is always important to check for a chip due to the fact that it can eventually spread into a crack across the entire surface of the lens.

Wrong prescription

This type of error is self explanatory. When neutralizing or reading a prescription in lenses with a lensmeter, automatic or manual, by ANSI standards, only a certain very small percentage of err is to be overlooked. If it goes over the documented ANSI standard, the eyewear must be rejected and the lenses re-cut.

Loose lens fit

Upon final inspection of mounted eyewear, the fit of the lens to the frame must be extremely snug so that the lenses will not move while mounted in the frame. Movement of lenses in eyewear will cause it to go off axis, thus, changing the overall prescription. The higher or more powerful the prescription, the less the axis can be moved.

Gaps in eyewear

Sometimes one will find what is called and looks like gaps in eyewear. That is because this is really what they are – gaps. There should be no gaps, or openings big or minute, between the lens and the frame at any point.

Uneven Bevels

Bevels are placed around the edges of the lenses during the fabrication process of edging using a machine called an edger. A different type of bevel is put on the back edges of the lenses to avoid scratching the patient's face. This other bevel, called a **safety bevel,** is done using the manual edger, or hand stone. When beveling a lens with the manual edger or hand stone, the bevels are supposed to be even and smooth all the way around the lens. They should not be too thick and barely noticeable. If the safety bevel is uneven and rough, the eyewear will fail inspection.

The bevel done on the automatic edger is used to create a secure hold for the lenses in frames. Care should be taken in placement of this bevel as prescription and type of frame need to be first considered before beginning the process. A bevel placed in the wrong area on the lens can result in a lens that continues to pop out of the frame.

Waves

This type of wave isn't the hello, bye-bye one. Instead it is the type of wave that can appear in the finishing product of a lens during the prefabrication, or first stages in making the prescription. If a lens is overheated, through the generating process or cylinder machine process, a wave will be formed inside the lens. This wave will alter the patient's vision if dispensed, therefore, care should be taken in locating waves.

Improper markings and blocking

If a lens is improperly marked or blocked, then the entire finished product will be canned. The marking and blocking errors can occur during the start or finish of a pair of lenses. Markings and blocking in the beginning will result in off axis errors, prism etc. Marking and blocking errors at the finish will result in pupillary distance errors, mounting issues etc. Therefore, when these type of errors occur, they are normally caught before dispensing. If not, the patient will automatically notice that something is terribly wrong. However, the eyewear shouldn't even make it to the patient when this occurs because the Optician should have inspected it and found these huge errors.

Contact Lenses Versus Eyeglasses – Advantages And Disadvantages

When it comes to selecting contact lenses versus eyeglasses, it's up to the particular individual's desires while they weigh the benefits and disadvantages to both contact lenses wear and eyeglasses. Both contact lenses and eyeglasses have advantages and disadvantages, and each patient will weigh those options carefully to make their own decision.

Below are some advantages to wearing eyeglasses over contact lenses:

- Cleaner to the eyeball, less likelihood of infection from not cleaning hands and contacts properly
- Requires less daily maintenance
- Less likely to gain corneal damage
- Can typically cost less than contacts over time
- Eyeglasses don't get stuck in the eyes, no trouble taking them off or putting on.

Now, below are some advantages to wearing contact lenses over eyeglasses:

- Great for sports (can wear safety glasses/shields if needed over contacts)
- Less peripheral distortion
- Overnight wear with many brands
- No irritating nose pads imprinting the face
- More compact
- Provides more hidden vision correction versus eyeglasses which are always obvious

According to my own experiences working with patients with **presbyopia**, most opted to use eyeglasses over contact lenses because many state poorer vision in bifocal or multi-focal contact lenses. Either these patients choose eyeglasses or opt for monovision contact lens wear.

What Are Bifocal Contact Lenses?

Bifocal contact lenses provide both near and distance vision for the patient, just the same as bifocal eyeglasses lenses, but only the bifocal contact lenses sit directly on the eyeball, or specifically, the cornea. Bifocal eyeglasses lenses sit in front of the eye, not touching the eyeball.

Despite the fact that bifocal contact lenses are made to perform similar to bifocal eyeglasses, the fact of the matter is that, after having worked with hundreds of patients, most prefer not to wear bifocal contact lenses after having given them a fair try. Bifocal contact lenses certain can create many setbacks like poorer vision than with glasses, thus, many times, a doctor will prescribe monovision wear.

Monovision contact lens wear is when an eye doctor prescribes for the **presbyopic** patient a near vision contact lens to wear in one eye. It has been my experience that presbyopic patients lean more toward this method. Other than that, many also opt to utilize near vision or bifocal glasses.

Interested in Becoming an Optician?

Becoming a certified or licensed Optician requires taking and passing the American Board of Opticianry Examinations given each year.

A high school graduate can become nationally certified if they pass national examination and is able to work anywhere in the United States with this national certification. However, in order to become a licensed Optician, one must pass the state board as well after a mandatory apprenticeship under a licensed Optician or gaining a formal education for the skill in school.

After becoming an Optician, every three years, one must complete several continuing education hours in order to renew the certification or licensing.

Visit the American Board of Opticianry online to get started on your journey to becoming an Optician.